# FAQs on Statistics
# in Clinical Trials

by
## Professor Andrew P Grieve

**BROOKWOOD MEDICAL PUBLICATIONS**

# ABOUT
# THE AUTHOR

Professor Andrew Grieve is the senior statistical consultant in the Biometrics Department at Pfizer Central Research, Sandwich, UK. He has spent more the 20 years in the pharmaceutical industry both in the UK and in Switzerland. His experience ranges from drug discovery, pre-clinical safety, and clinical development to pharmaceutical development and production. He is a keen advocate of the use of Bayesian statistics in drug development. He has served on the Council of the Royal Statistical Society and is currently chairperson of Statisticians in the Pharmaceutical Industry.

# CONTENTS

## Preface

Statisticians and clinicians who work together to develop new drugs or surgical techniques need to communicate with one another. Communication difficulties often arise through a lack of understanding of the scientific languages used by different parties. Each side has a responsibility to improve understanding. Statisticians must become familiar with the medical viewpoint while clinicians need to have a broad understanding of the underlying principles of good statistical practice.

At the end of the twentieth century it would be nice to think that William Osler's words "Medicine will become a science when doctors learn to count" are no longer as true as they once were. However Wulff et al[1] concluded in a recent report that "the statistical knowledge of most doctors is so limited that they cannot be expected to draw the right conclusions from those statistical analyses which are found in papers in medical journals".

This book is aimed at promoting a better understanding by clinicians of some of the most common statistical issues. The issues selected in this book are those which I have found to be of common interest to the clinicians with whom I have worked during my twenty years in the pharmaceutical industry. Clearly any such choice is personal, and subjective, and it is not my intention to provide exhaustive coverage of statistical issues which might possibly be of interest to clinicians. The topics included range from the basic principles, such as appropriate uses of means, modes and medians, to the highly complex ideas underlying Bayesian statistics.

I would welcome comments from clinicians regarding the issues in this book they feel are of most relevance to them in their daily practice. But, more importantly, I would like to hear about those issues, of equal interest and concern, which I have not covered. I therefore invite anybody who has such questions to complete the form on page 59 and return it to the address given, in order that I may endeavour to provide an answer.

A P Grieve

# 1

## Basic Statistical Concepts

## *Q* Why do we need statistics in drug development?

In the last twenty years there has been a rapid growth in the numbers of statisticians employed globally in the drug development industry, and this is also true in the United Kingdom. The membership of the British organisation "Statisticians in the Pharmaceuticals Industry" has grown from 50 members in 1977 to over 800 today (see figure 1). Why?

**Figure 1:** *Membership of PSI 1977-1997*

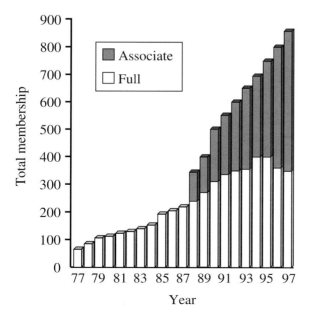

Although it could be claimed that the increase is due to a realisation by clinical and non-clinical researchers alike that statisticians have much to offer, in fact the growth is a direct consequence of increased governmental regulation of the drug development process. Newly-established regulations include those governing Good Laboratory Practice (GLP) which controls the use of animal experiments and toxicology studies, Good Clinical Practice (GCP) which regulates human experimentation, and Good Manufacturing Practice (GMP) which regulates the pharmaceutical manufacturing processes. Each of these regulations recognises the importance of three critical aspects of the role of statisticians: design, analysis and reporting.

While many scientists may employ a statistician at the analysis and reporting stages of a project, most statisticians would argue that their most important contribution can be made in the design phase. Good design is crucial if reliable inferences are to made from experimental data. Good design ensures that problems of bias are minimised, that wastage of scarce experimental resources is kept to a minimum and hence that drug development is carried out more efficiently. As Sir Ronald Fisher, the father of modern statistics, said:

*"To call in the statistician after the experiment is done may be no more than asking him to perform a post-mortem examination: he may be able to say what the experiment died of."*

# *Q*  What is the difference between the median, the mode and the mean?

**The mean of a sample of values is the arithmetic average and is determined by dividing the sum of the values by the number of values.**

For example the following are 50 values of the Ritchie Index, a measure of joint stiffness in patients with rheumatoid arthritis, taken from untreated patients[2]:

14 9 8 9 1 20 3 3 2 4 2 3 6 1 2 11 16 24 16 21 19 22 33 12
12 12 19 10 33 2 19 40 1 20 1 2 4 7 9 4 9 6 14 8 27 10 27 7 24 21

Their arithmetic mean is:

$$\text{mean} = \frac{14+9+8+ ...+24+21}{50} = \frac{609}{50} = 12.18$$

**The median is the typical value. It is the midpoint of the values when they are arranged in ascending order (if there are an even number of values there is no midpoint value and the average of the two middle values is taken).**

In ascending order the Ritchie Index values are

1 1 1 1 2 2 2 2 2 3 3 3 4 4 4 6 6 7 7 8 8 9 9 9 9 <u>9 10</u> 10 11
12 12 12 14 14 16 16 19 19 19 20 20 21 21 22 24 24 27 27 33 33 40

and the median is the average of the 25th and 26th values:

$$\text{median} = \frac{9 + 10}{2} = 9.5$$

**The mode is the most frequently-occurring value.**

The mode of the Ritchie Index values is 2 because this value occurs five times and no other value appears more than four times.

Each of these measures is intended in some sense to be representative of the sample as a whole. To what extent are they successful?

**Figure 2:** *Histogram of Ritchie Index values from a sample of 50 untreated patients*

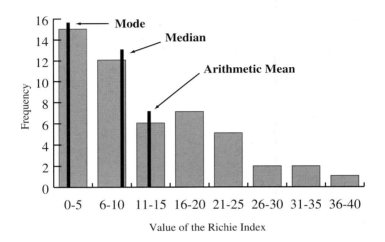

The **mode** is little used as a summary of data because it records only the most frequent value, which may be far from the centre of the distribution of values. Indeed this is true for our example (see Figure 2) in which the sample mode is on the extreme left of the histogram. A second problem is that there can be more than one mode in a sample. For example, if one of the 2s above had been missing then not only 2, but also 1 and 9 would be modes of the remaining 49 values. The mode has the unique advantage that it may be used for characteristics which are measured on a nominal scale. For example, the most frequent, or modal, gender of a sample has a meaning unlike the mean or the median gender.

The **median** does not use the actual numerical values; instead it uses the relative size of the values. It can therefore be used for data recorded in categories (e.g. absent, mild, moderate, severe) as well as for interval data (e.g. temperature, blood pressure). The median is not affected by extreme values far from the centre, for example the median of 49 old age pensioners and one new-born infant gives the age of the vast majority and is unaffected by the extreme value.

The **mean** utilises the most information in the data because it relies on the actual numerical values, and is the most commonly used measure of the centre of a distribution. In strict terms, it should only be used for variables which are recorded as interval data. However it is often applied inappropriately to data in which the categories are arbitrarily assigned numerical values, for example: 1=absent, 2=mild, 3=moderate, 4=severe. In taking an average over such categories we make an implicit assumption that a change from absent to mild is the same as a change from moderate to severe.

The appropriate measure to use depends on the context; there is no single measure which will be correct in all circumstances.

# *Q* What are the geometric and harmonic means and when should they be used?

Consider the following example. An intravenous administration of 2 µg/kg of lysergic acid diethylamide (LSD) to 5 normal human subjects gave the following mean plasma concentrations as a function of time after administration:

| Time (minutes) | 10 | 30 | 60 | 120 | 240 | 480 |
|---|---|---|---|---|---|---|
| Concentration (µg/litre) | 9.5 | 6.3 | 5.3 | 4.2 | 2.9 | 1.2 |

What is an estimate of the concentration after 20 minutes?

In this instance the arithmetic mean of 9.5 µg/litre and 6.3 µg/litre, i.e. the values after 10 and 30 minutes, is not a good estimate because it assumes that the concentration decreases by a constant amount in a given time interval. The arithmetic mean is 7.9 µg/litre, which is 1.6 µg/litre less than 9.5 µg/litre and 1.6 µg/litre greater than 6.3 µg/litre. However it is more usual to assume that the plasma concentration decreases at a constant rate, in other words the concentration decreases by a proportionate amount in a given time interval. In such cases an "average" based upon multiplication rather than addition is appropriate. This is the **geometric mean**.

**Figure 3:** *Mean concentration/time profile of 5 subjects following administration of 2µg/kg of LSD*

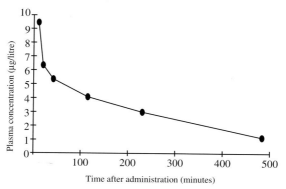

If we remember that the arithmetic mean was arrived at by adding all the values together and dividing by n (the number of values), the geometric mean has a similar structure.

> **The geometric mean of a sample of n values is determined by multiplying all the values together and taking the nth root (for only two values this is the more familiar square root).**

So for the LSD concentration at 20 minutes a more appropriate estimate is given by $\sqrt{9.5 \times 6.3} = 7.7$ µg/litre. There is little difference between these two estimates because in that part of the data the decline is approximately linear (see Figure 3). However it can be seen from this figure that if one was to use the arithmetic mean over the whole range, a considerable error could arise. For example the arithmetic average of the values recorded after 10 and 480 minutes is 5.35 µg/litre while the geometric average is $\sqrt{9.5 \times 1.2} = 3.38$ µg/litre. This latter value is reasonably close to the value of 2.9 µg/litre observed at 240 minutes.

Consider the following example. A study is conducted to investigate the effect of a treatment on epileptic patients. Five patients are studied and the time in weeks to the occurrence of 20 attacks is recorded. The individual attack rates are as follows (per week):

**1.82  1.33  2.22  1.67  0.83.**

What is the average attack rate? The obvious answer is $(1.82+1.33+2.22+1.67+0.83)/5 = 1.57$ attacks/week. This is wrong because it averages the number of attacks as a function of time, but the time element is different for each individual. It is more appropriate to average the different time elements to achieve a given number of attacks and to convert this into an attack rate per unit time. This may be achieved directly by calculating the **harmonic mean** of the individual attack rates.

> **The harmonic mean of a sample of n values is determined by summing the reciprocals of all the values and dividing this sum into n.**

For the attack rates above the harmonic mean is given by:

$$\frac{5}{\frac{1}{1.82} + \frac{1}{1.33} + \frac{1}{2.22} + \frac{1}{1.67} + \frac{1}{0.83}} = 1.14 \text{ attacks/week}$$

In medical applications, cases requiring such analyses rarely arise. This is because more often than not time is fixed and the occurrence of events is variable. For example, when investigating antiepileptic therapies a study might last for three months and the number of attacks in the three month period would be of prime interest.

There are some circumstances in which the harmonic mean is implicitly used. It is sometimes necessary when using standard statistical techniques, such as the t-test or analysis of variance, to transform the data in order that the assumptions of the methods are more closely met. For example, many statisticians would say that before analysing heart rate data the reciprocal of the heart rates should be analysed rather than heart rates themselves. The resulting variable is the duration of a heart beat. If the resulting mean heart beat duration is itself reciprocated the resulting average heart rate is the harmonic mean of the original rates.

# *Q* How is the variability of a sample of values measured?

In the previous questions we examined methods of summarising some aspect of the "average" value within a sample. A second important characteristic of a sample is its variability.

Suppose a new production process for the manufacture of aspirin tablets has been developed. The tablets are to have a nominal content of 100 mg. A random sample of tablets from the new process is assayed and has the following measured contents (mg):

**96  97  100  101  101**

The mean of these values is 99 mg. A second sample from the old process is also assayed and gives the following results (mg):

**88  93  100  104  110**

Again the mean content is 99 mg. Although the mean values are identical, the new process is better because the contents are less variable than those produced by the old process, i.e. the processes differ in the amount of spread or variability.

**Figure 4:** *Inter-quartile range of a sample of 50 Ritchie Index values of untreated patients*

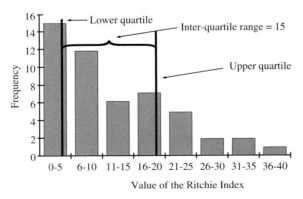

Defining formal measures of spread allows us to compare different data for this characteristic. There are a number of measures of spread which are commonly used.

The **range** of a set of data is defined as the largest value minus the smallest value. For the two samples above the ranges are 5 mg for the new process and 22 mg for the old process. Although the range is an extremely simple statistic to calculate it has two major disadvantages. First, it uses only the maximum and minimum values and ignores the rest of the data. Second, as the number of values in the sample increases, in general so does the range.

The **inter-quartile range** is a second measure of dispersion and is based on the **quartiles** of the data. The lower quartile is that value which is greater than one quarter of the data, and less than three quarters of the data; similarly, the upper quartile is that value which is greater than three quarters of the data, and less than one quarter of the data. The inter-quartile range is the difference between the two.

Example: determine the inter-quartile range of the Ritchie Index values introduced on page 7.

The lower quartile of the 50 values is that value which is greater than 12.5 (i.e. 50/4) values. Similarly, the upper quartile is that value which is less than 12.5 values. The former is half-way between the 13th and 14th values, while the latter is half-way between the 37th and 38th values. Look at the ordered Ritchie values:

**1 1 1 1 2 2 2 2 2 2 3 3 3 4 4 4 6 6 7 7 8 8 9 9 9 9 10 10 11 12 12 12 14 14 16 16 19 19 19 20 20 21 21 22 24 24 27 27 33 33 40**

The lower and upper quartiles are 4 and 19 respectively, giving an inter-quartile range of 15. In Figure 4 the upper and lower quartiles of the data are shown. These values contain 50% of the values in the sample.

These two measures do not take account of the numerical values recorded; they only use the relative magnitudes. The **standard deviation** is a measure which accounts for the magnitudes and determines an average amount by which values in the sample differ from the sample mean. To illustrate its calculation consider again the contents (mg) from the new aspirin production process:

**96  97  100  101  101  (mean 99 mg)**

Next we determine the deviations of the individual values from the mean :

**-3  -2  1  2  2**

It is meaningless to calculate the average of these deviations because their sum, by definition, is zero. Instead we square them to make them all positive, sum these values and calculate the average. The square root of this is the standard deviation.

$$\text{Standard deviation} = \sqrt{\frac{9 + 4 + 1 + 4 + 4}{5}} = 4.4$$

(More properly the sum of squared deviations is divided not by n but by n-1.)

# *Q* What is the difference between the standard error and the standard deviation?

In the previous question we considered measures of variability associated with a sample. While the variability of a sample may be of interest, particularly when we wish to determine the size of a new study, in many cases we are more interested in the variability of a statistic or a summary measure calculated from the population, such as the mean. In order to understand how the variability of the mean taken from a population differs from the variability of the values in the population we will carry out a sampling experiment using the Ritchie Index values introduced on page 7.

The sampling experiment was done by randomly selecting measurements from the original 50, calculating their means and repeating the process a number of times. 50 random samples of 10 observations were taken from the 50 values of the Ritchie index. The end-point of this process is a series of 50 means, which are not all equal, so that they themselves show random variation. There are a large number of possible ways to choose 10 values out of 50, and the 50 which we have determined is a random sample from the so-called **sampling distribution** of the mean.

**Figure 5:** *Histogram of random samples of means of size 10 from original population of 50 patients*

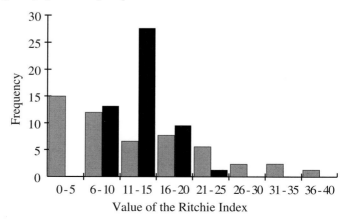

Because the 50 means are themselves a random sample from a distribution we can determine certain properties of that distribution, such as the mean and the standard deviation. The mean of the mean is 12.21 and the standard deviation is 2.97. The mean of the population of values is 12.18, close to the mean of the sample means. However the standard deviation of the population of values is 9.69, which is considerably larger than that of the sample of means. This is indicative of the sample means being less variable than individual values from the population. Figure 5 is a histogram of the sample means which has been superimposed on the original histogram of individual values:

> **The standard deviation of the sampling distribution of the mean is called the standard error of the mean.**

We saw that the sampling variation of the mean of samples is less than the variation of the individual values. This reduction in variability depends on the sample size on which the means are based. For example, if the means are based on 20 values a similar sampling experiment gives a standard deviation of the means of 2.10. In other words the sample size has an important influence on the standard error.

**Figure 6:** *Standard error of the mean as a function of the sample size*

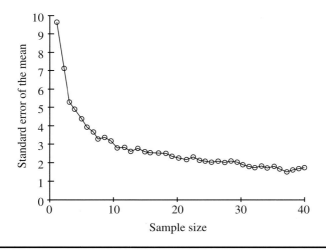

Figure 6 shows the relationship between the standard error of the mean and the sample size estimated from a further sampling experiment. The precise relationship which this figure reflects is that if the population standard deviation is $\sigma$, the standard error is $\sigma / \sqrt{n}$.

The difference between these two concepts is very important and must be clarified. The mean is often seen in reports written as, for example, $12.18 \pm 1.37$, and it is unclear whether 1.37 refers to the standard error or the standard deviation.

# *Q* What confidence can we have in a confidence interval?

The mean Ritchie Index is a single value and is known as a **point estimate**. It is extremely unlikely that the mean of a sample of values is exactly the same as the population mean of which it is an estimate. The sample mean may be close to the population mean, and the amount by which it is most likely to differ from the population mean is determined by the standard error. In order to formally acknowledge the uncertainty in such an estimate it is usual to determine an **interval estimate**. An interval estimate is a pair of values for the parameter within which the population parameter is likely to lie. The most common form of interval estimate is the **confidence interval**.

When using a population mean, the 95% confidence interval for the population mean is approximated by:

sample mean  ± 1.96 x standard error

We have seen that the mean and standard error of the original 50 values of the Ritchie index are 12.18 and 1.37 respectively, so that approximately 95% confidence limits for the population mean are:

12.18 ± 1.96 x 1.37 = 9.49 – 14.87

But in what sense can we be 95% confident that the population mean lies within the limits 9.49 and 14.87? In order to answer this question we can again conduct a sampling experiment.

As before, suppose that 50 values comprise the whole population, and that the sampling experiment again consists of randomly selecting 10 observations from the 50. In this instance the mean, standard error and the 95% confidence interval for the mean are determined. The sampling is then repeated 100 times. The results of these calculations is illustrated in Figure 7.

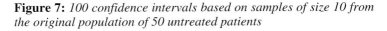

**Figure 7:** *100 confidence intervals based on samples of size 10 from the original population of 50 untreated patients*

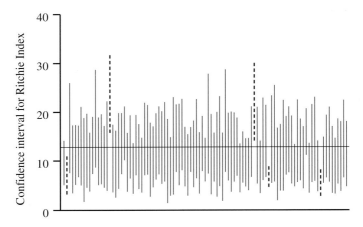

In this figure the confidence interval for each of the 100 samples is drawn as a vertical line between the lower and upper limits. The horizontal reference line is positioned at the population mean of 12.18. What can we say about the 100 confidence intervals? Clearly the vast majority are close to the population value; in fact 95 of the 100 intervals include within them the population value, and only 5 (shown as dotted lines) do not. So 95% of the intervals contain the true value. Here then is the basis of our confidence. It is confidence based upon the idea of being able to repeat the sampling, and the calculation.

Confidence intervals are not restricted to statements about mean values. For example, Braitman[3] considers an estimate of the proportion of patients showing complete response to treatment for ovarian cancer. In the following extract Braitman describes the confidence we can have in a confidence interval as follows :

*"The proper interpretation of confidence intervals requires that we consider a large number of hypothetical random samples (each of the same size). Then '95% confidence' means that approximately 95% of the 95% confidence intervals from these random samples*

*would include the unknown true value, and about 5% would not. Because the true fraction in the population is unknown, it is impossible to tell if the 95% confidence interval of 28% to 55% that was obtained from the observed sample data actually includes the true fraction. Strictly speaking, we cannot even tell how likely the 95% confidence interval of 28% to 55% is to include the unknown true fraction. Nevertheless, the usual interpretation is that we are 95% confident that the unknown true value is between 28% and 55%."*

In essence the probabilities (95% or other levels) involved in confidence intervals are probabilities concerning the procedure for calculating the intervals.

There is debate among statisticians regarding the appropriateness of confidence intervals. The problem is that the "usual interpretation" referred to by Braitman, although not supported by the confidence interval procedure, is precisely the form of statement that many users of confidence intervals would like to make. The "usual interpretation" is supported by a different approach to statistics called Bayesian statistics, which is discussed on page 53.

There has been a movement over the last 15 years to usurp the position of p-values (see page 22) from their position of pre-eminence in clinical trials. The campaign culminated in the publication of a book dedicated to the confidence interval, published under the auspices of the British Medical Journal[4]. This book provides many examples of confidence intervals for a wide variety of parameters. These include, for example, the relative risk and the odds ratio – see page 31.

# *Q* What is a p-value and is it different from a significance level?

Much of what has been considered up to this point has been concerned with estimation. However, the type of statistical inference more often used in medical data is significance testing. To illustrate the basic idea of significance testing we will use the data shown in Table 1. The data are taken from a crossover experiment (see page 26) in which 20 patients were each given an active treatment and a placebo to treat severe headaches. The primary response outcome was the proportion of days on which a headache occurred, over a time period varying between 42 and 64 days. The objective of the trial was to show that the new treatment reduced the proportion of days on which headaches occurred. Table 1 shows the proportion of days with headache on which the active drug and placebo were given,

**Table 1:** *Data from a crossover experiment – proportion of days with a headache*

| Placebo | Active | Difference | Sign of Difference |
|---------|--------|------------|--------------------|
| 0.68 | 0.61 | 0.07 | + |
| 0.96 | 1.00 | -0.04 | - |
| 0.85 | 0.72 | 0.13 | + |
| 0.93 | 0.81 | 0.12 | + |
| 0.35 | 0.26 | 0.09 | + |
| 0.77 | 0.70 | 0.07 | + |
| 0.74 | 0.61 | 0.13 | + |
| 0.98 | 1.00 | -0.02 | - |
| 1.00 | 0.98 | 0.02 | + |
| 0.28 | 0.16 | 0.12 | + |
| 0.92 | 0.79 | 0.13 | + |
| 1.00 | 0.98 | 0.02 | + |
| 0.93 | 1.00 | -0.07 | - |
| 1.00 | 0.96 | 0.04 | + |
| 0.45 | 0.49 | -0.04 | - |
| 0.82 | 0.74 | 0.08 | + |
| 0.36 | 0.26 | 0.10 | + |
| 1.00 | 0.97 | 0.03 | + |
| 0.49 | 0.43 | 0.06 | + |
| 0.74 | 0.66 | 0.08 | + |

as well as the difference in proportions (placebo-active) and whether the difference is positive or negative.

To carry out a test of significance we suppose that there is no difference between the treatments, i.e. the null hypothesis. This **null hypothesis** is tested against an **alternative hypothesis** which says that there is a difference between the treatments, and the difference can be in either direction, active is better than placebo or placebo is better than active. If the null hypothesis is true then we would expect to see as many plusses as minuses, i.e. probability that the difference is positive = probability that the difference is negative = 0.5

Since there are 20 patients the distribution of the number of plusses and minuses will be a **binomial distribution** with parameters $n = 20$ and $p = 0.5$ and we would expect to see $np = 10$ minuses. The binomial distribution has the property that the probability of r out n outcomes is given by:

$$\frac{n!}{r!(n - r)!} \, p^r \, (1 - p)^{n-r} \qquad \text{where } r = 0,1,2....n$$

From Table 1 it can be seen that there are 4 minuses out of 20 outcomes. Given that there is no difference between the treatments the probability of this result is:

$$\frac{20}{4!16!} \, 0.5^4 \, 0.5^{16} = 4845 \times 0.5^{20} = 0.00462$$

Taken in isolation, this is not an unlikely event. However in significance testing we are estimating the likelihood of an event which is at least as far from what is expected as the observed value. Figure 8 shows the entire binomial distribution; it can be seen that the values $r = 3,2,1,0$ are all at least as extreme as the observed value of 4. Similar calculations show that these events have probabilities of 0.00109, 0.00018, 0.00002 and 0.000001 respectively. Thus the probability of 4 or fewer minuses is the sum of these values, which equals 0.0059.

**Figure 8:** *Distribution of the number of minuses out of 20 given that there is no difference between the treatments*

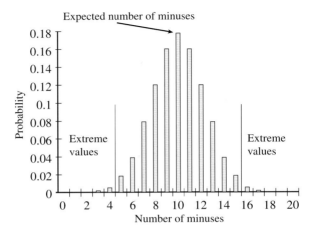

Because we are interested in alternatives in both directions we need to consider values as far from the expected in the other direction. It is clear from Figure 8 that the distribution is symmetrical and therefore we are interested in the values 16,17,18,19 and 20. The sum of probabilities for each of these events is the same as we have already calculated, i.e. 0.0059. Hence the probability of getting as extreme a value, in either direction, is 2 x 0.0059 = 0.0118. This is the **p-value.**

> **The p-value is the probability of observing a value at least as large as was observed if the null hypothesis is true.**

The p-value in this example is quite small and therefore we have observed an extremely unlikely event if there was no difference between the treatments. Thus the data are not consistent with the null hypothesis and we may conclude that there is strong evidence that the active treatments reduces the incidence of headache days compared to placebo.

What does small mean? If the probability above had been 0.04 or 0.12 would we have felt the same strength in a conclusion that the treatments are different? Many people use 0.05 as a standard level below which they are prepared to conclude the null hypothesis is false. If we were to do that then if the null hypothesis were true 5 times out of 100 we would conclude that the null hypothesis was false. Deciding against a true null hypothesis is termed an error of the first kind and the probability of making such an error is called the **type-I error** or **significance level.**

# 2

## Design Issues

*Q* **Why are crossover designs not universally appropriate?**

The use of a crossover design in which each patient receives more than one of the treatments under test has an intuitive appeal to clinicians. The design has three fundamental advantages:

1      In such designs individual patients act as their own control, so that the different treatments are compared within individual patients.

2      A direct consequence of the patient acting as their own control is that, because in general there is less variability within patients than between patients, the comparison of treatments will be more precise. This has two important implications: it is economical, because in order to achieve a certain sensitivity in comparing treatments fewer patients will be required in a crossover design than in a parallel group design; and ethically in that fewer patients will be exposed to the danger of an ineffective treatment or to adverse events.

3      In a crossover design individual patients, or the clinicians, are able to express a direct preference for one treatment, or the other.

However, crossover designs have one substantial drawback, which is that they require assumptions to be made in order to avoid bias, as Bradford-Hill[5] pointed out:

*"In some instances it may be better to design the trial so that each patient provides his own control, by having various treatments in turn. This is known as a crossover trial... By such means we may sometimes make the comparison more sensitive since we have*

*eliminated the variability that must exist between patients treated at the same stage of the disease in question (so far as can be judged). We have done so, however, at the expense of introducing as a factor the variability within patients from one time to another, i.e. we may be giving the patient treatment A and treatment B at different stages of the disease."*

The possibility of treating patients at different stages of their disease causes problems in the use of crossover trials. An obvious way in which this might happen is if one, or both, of the treatments is curative. If both are curative then there is no point in using a crossover study; if one is curative and the other not then the position at the start of the second treatment is inequitable because patients who received the curative treatment in the first treatment period no longer have the disease and therefore for these individuals the other treatment appears to be equally effective. This is an extreme form of what is termed "**carryover**", i.e. the idea that the effect of a treatment taken in the first period may persist into the second period. In theory the presence of carryover can cause serious bias to treatment estimates. There are a number of causes of carryover[6]:

- It is of particular importance when designing a crossover trial to ensure that there is an adequate washout period between the two treatment periods. Failure to ensure this may result in a pharmacological carryover.

- Treatment in the first period may cause a change to the patient's physiological or psychological state. For example, an active treatment may be so potent that the patient is functionally unblinded, i.e. they know the treatment they have received and are therefore predisposed to expect little from the treatment in the second period.

- The treatment effect may depend on the individual patient disease severity. This can usually be removed by the appropriate choice of transformation.

- There may be a period-by-treatment interaction, in which the difference between treatments differs from period-to-period.

- There may be a general difference between the average patient effects in the two sequence randomisation groups.

Although there is a test for carryover, the potential causes are indistinguishable in the statistical model. Indeed, it is possible to contemplate more than one of these being present in any particular trial. There are four standard approaches to analysing crossover trials, in particular to handling potential carryover:

- In the first approach no thought is given to the potential for pharmacological or psychological carryover. In particular the likely lengths of the drug half-life or washout period are not considered. The data are analysed ignoring the possibility of a carryover.

- In the second approach it is assumed that there is always the possibility of a carryover of a size which could bias treatment estimates. Although a preliminary test for carryover exists, it is known to be insensitive and therefore unreliable. Adherents of this approach tend not to recommend crossover designs.

- The third approach requires that a preliminary test for carryover be performed. Depending on the result of the test, an analysis ignoring the possibility of carryover is carried out (preliminary test non-significant) or the data from the second period are ignored because they are regarded as unreliable and the first period data are analysed as if they had arisen from a parallel group design (preliminary test significant). This approach is known to have very bad statistical properties[7].

- In the last approach the possibility of carryover is always considered. The question is asked "can an adequate washout be utilised to avoid carryover?" If it can then a crossover trial can be designed and analysed ignoring carryover. If it cannot then a crossover trial should not be used.

# $Q$ Why must we use concurrent randomised controls?

The use of concurrent, randomised, controls in experimental science is essential in order to ensure that observed effects are real. In order to understand this we will consider other forms of controls whose use is not recommended.

## *Concurrent, non-randomised controls*

Suppose a doctor decides to conduct an experiment in his surgery: he prescribes a given dose of a drug to some patients with the target disease, to others he does not. The progress of the patients is monitored over time and at some appropriate juncture the results of the two groups of patients are compared. In order for this comparison to be valid it is necessary to assume that the two groups of patients are identical in all respects relevant to their disease and its progress. Without the use of randomisation it is incorrect to make such an assumption. Why? The doctor may be tempted to allocate the drug to certain patients on the basis of the severity of the condition. It is therefore possible that the most severe patients are given the new drug while the less severe patients are not. Hence it is difficult to come to a conclusion about the potential effects of the drug. Even in those cases where such an overtly biased allocation does not occur, without randomisation other less subtle biases cannot be prevented.

## *The patient as their own control*

Except in the special circumstances in which a crossover design can be used, the use of the patient as their own control is not appropriate (see page 26). In such studies - sometimes labelled "before-and-after" or "pretest-posttest" designs - there are no concurrent randomised controls, and the comparison is made between the pre-treatment and post-treatment disease severities. Such designs make two assumptions:

i       that there are no changes in the conditions between the two occasions on which measurements are taken, for example, measuring the severity of hayfever during the summer followed by treatment and measurement of the severity for a second time in the autumn;

ii      that there is not a natural progression of the disease over time, for example, the observation that if you treat a cold it lasts for a week, if you do not it lasts seven days.

*Historical controls*

The use of historical controls involves the comparison of data taken from previously untreated patients with currently treated patients. For example, suppose that in a series of previously untreated patients 20% died and 80% survived, while in the current series 5% died and 95% survived. Is it valid to conclude that the new treatment is effective? First we need to be able to assume that the groups of patients are essentially similar in every respect but their treatment. We need to be certain that the demographic profiles of the patients were the same, that the disease severities were the same and that there was no essential change to the way in which patients were handled. To be sure of all these factors is extremely difficult; indeed we can only be sure that they are similar with respect to characteristics which have been measured and recorded. Randomisation protects against lack of balance with respect to those characteristics which are measured, as well as those which are not.

Despite the above arguments there are circumstances in which it may not be possible to use concurrent, randomised controls. Suppose for example that a disease is almost always fatal and that the death occurs quickly. In such circumstances there is no need to have concurrent controls to show that there has been a change in the death rate. There may also be ethical difficulties in justifying the withholding of a treatment which it is believed to be beneficial in such acute diseases.

# Advanced Topics

*Q* **Which is more appropriate: difference in proportions, relative risk or odds ratio?**

The data in Table 2 are typical of many clinical trials, in that they compare two treatments (inoculation versus control) and record whether patients develop typhoid infection or not. The data are taken from a meta-analysis which is discussed on page 48. The basic building blocks of any inference about the difference between the effects of the two treatments which may be made upon such data are the observed rates, or proportion of infected patients.

**Table 2:** *Effect of inoculation on the incidence of typhoid infection*

| Treatment | Infected | Not Infected | Total |
|-----------|----------|--------------|-------|
| Inoculated | 11 | 76 | 87 |
| Control | 13 | 34 | 47 |

In this example the incidence of typhoid amongst those inoculated is $11/87 = 12.6\%$, while the corresponding rate amongst controls is $13/47 = 27.7\%$. These observed rates are estimates of the population incidence rates, $\pi_I$ for inoculated and $\pi_C$ for controls. Any representation of differences between the treatments will be based upon these population rates.

There are three main approaches to representing treatment differences, each of which would normally be presented together with an associated confidence interval (see page 19):

1  The simplest approach looks at the difference between the rates: $\delta = \pi_C - \pi_I$ Thus in the example in Table 2 the estimated absolute rate reduction (**ARR**) is $27.7 - 12.6 = 15.1\%$.

2      A second approach looks at the ratio of the rates: $\phi = \pi_C - \pi_I$. For the typhoid data the estimated relative risk (**RR**) is $0.277/0.216 = 2.19$, in other words the risk of becoming infected with typhoid among controls is approximately twice that among those inoculated.

3      The final approach looks at the odds ratio (**OR**): $\theta = \pi_C(1-\pi_I)/[\pi_I(1-\pi_C)]$. For the typhoid data the estimated odds ratio is $0.126 \times 0.723/(0.874 \times 0.277) = 2.66$.

Two major issues differentiate between the three measures: relative versus absolute effects and understandability.

The RR is the simplest of the two measures and provides a measure of the relative size of difference in event rates between two groups, but does not give any indication of either the level of the effect of the absolute difference between groups. For example:

Case 1:    $\pi_C = 0.02$, $\pi_I = 0.01$
Case 2:    $\pi_C = 0.40$, $\pi_I = 0.20$

Both cases give an RR of 2 and yet are very different, with Case 2 likely to be more clinically important than Case 1. The latter measure is the converse, for example:

Case 3:    $\pi_C = 0.20$, $\pi_I = 0.10$
Case 4:    $\pi_C = 0.70$, $\pi_I = 0.60$

Cases 3 and 4 both give an ARR of 0.10 but again are very different, this time Case 3 is probably clinically more interesting than Case 4.

It is difficult to provide a hard and fast rule as to which of these two measures is the best. Studies have shown that choice of measure can have an important influence on clinical judgement and subsequent management of a patient; given that there is a degree of complementarity between the two measures, perhaps both should be presented.

The odds ratio is an alternative to the RR as a relative measure. From examining the form of the odds ratio below, it should be clear that if the individual risks are low, the OR and the RR are approximately equal. This can cause some confusion and at times the terms are used interchangeably.

$$OR = \frac{\pi_C}{\pi_I} \frac{1 - \pi_I}{1 - \pi_C} = RR \times \frac{1 - \pi_I}{1 - \pi_C}$$

There appears to be a widespread inability or unwillingness to understand the OR. Most lay people only encounter odds in the realm of horse-racing, for example Red Rum is 5-to-1 against winning the Grand National, Desert Orchid is 2-to-1 on to win the Cheltenham Gold Cup. Ratios of such concepts are not easy to grasp and are not intuitively meaningful and yet the OR has become pervasive in the meta-analysis literature (see page 48). Why? The main reason is the simplicity of the statistical analysis of the odds ratio compared to RR, which was a major consideration before the advent of computer analysis. Simplicity is no longer a sine qua non for a statistical method, and computer analyses are readily available for most of the analyses. It is likely, therefore, that the OR will lose its position of predominance in the area of meta-analysis.

# $Q$   What is the NNT?

In the previous question we concluded that the RR and the ARR provide complementary information and that in the future the OR is likely to be used less often. An alternative measure was introduced by Laupacis et al[8] in order to facilitate interpretation in terms of patients treated rather than the less intuitively understandable probabilities, and even less intuitively understandable OR.

> **The number needed to treat (NNT) is the number of patients which it is necessary to treat before one "adverse" event is prevented. It is related to the absolute risk reduction (see page 31) by:**
>
> $$NNT = \frac{1}{ARR}$$

Applying this idea to the data in Table 2 we have:

$$NNT = \frac{1}{0.277 - 0.126} = 6.66$$

The interpretation of this result is that one typhoid infection was prevented for every 7 patients treated. As with other statistics this is merely an estimate of the true NNT and it is appropriate to report it together with an associated confidence interval. This may be determined by inverting the confidence interval for the ARR.

Because the NNT is directly related to the ARR there is little extra advantage in its use. However the expression of the NNT in terms of number of patients who have to be treated before some benefit accrues is believed, at least by disciples of the NNT, to facilitate interpretation rather than what are seen as less intuitive probabilities, or proportions. It is almost certainly true that individuals who are comfortable with numeric data will find little use for the NNT. However there will be those who will find the NNT an attractive alternative to the ARR, RR and especially the OR.

**If the difference between treatments is not significant, why aren't the treatments equal?**

The data in Table 3 are taken from the meta-analysis on page 48. To analyse these data we could either carry out a significance test, associated with the null hypothesis that the infection rates amongst inoculated patients and controls are the same, or we can estimate a parameter such as the RR and provide an interval estimate based on a confidence interval.

**Table 3:** *Effect of inoculation on the incidence of typhoid infection*

| Treatment | Infected | Not Infected | Total |
|-----------|----------|--------------|-------|
| Inoculated | 11 | 76 | 87 |
| Control | 13 | 34 | 47 |

*Significance Test*

There are a number of tests of significance associated with a test of the null hypothesis $H_0$: $\pi_C = \pi_I$ but probably the most common is the chi-squared test. For the data in Table 3 the chi-squared test gives a two-sided p-value of 0.894 and this value provides insufficient evidence to reject the null hypothesis.

*Confidence interval*

The estimated infection rates are 0.250 for inoculated patients and 0.231 for controls; therefore the estimated RR is 0.250/0.231 = 1.083 and its associated 95% confidence interval is 0.332 – 3.532. The width of the confidence interval explains why we are not justified in concluding that the treatments are the same just because they are not statistically significantly different. The narrow confidence interval shows that we are unable to reject the possibility that there are large differences between the treatments - a RR of over three might imply a great benefit for inoculation versus control.

A similar problem arises in adverse event reporting.[9] If a surgeon conducts a series of 10 operations and no patients suffer post-operative infections, is the surgeon justified in asserting that there is no danger of infection from the operation? The 95% confidence interval for the unknown infection rate is 0 - 0.26, i.e. the infection rate may be as high as one quarter. It is important to remember that absence of evidence is not evidence of absence![10] Another example of this mistake is the assumption implicitly shown on page 26 that a negative preliminary test for a carryover effect in a crossover trial implies that the main analysis of treatment effects may be conducted as if there was no carryover effect at all.

If the objective of a study is to show that there is no effective difference between two treatments then it is termed an **equivalence study**. The definition of what constitutes no effective difference needs to be determined before the study commences. Issues in designing and analysing equivalence studies are covered in a paper by Jones et al[11].

# *Q*   When adjusting for baseline which is preferable: analysis of covariance or change from baseline?

The data in Figure 9 are taken from a paper by Rikkers et al[12] which reported the results of a study examining the effect of a splenal shunt in cirrhotic patients. The study took the form of a comparative pre-test, post-test design in which the response variable (maximum rate of urea synthesis - MRUS) was measured before and after treatment. Should the baseline measurement be accounted for by analysis of covariance (ANCOVA) or by determining the change from baseline?

**Figure 9:** *MRUS data (from Rikkers et al)*

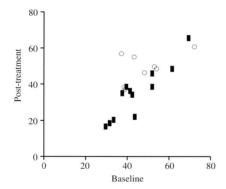

In order to choose between the two approaches we need to be aware of two issues:

1    What question(s) is answered by each approach and are they appropriate and/or different?

2    What assumption need to be made, and are they appropriate?

To address the first question consider the following paradox devised by Lord.[13] At the beginning and end of the academic year a university records the weights of all students who regularly eat meals in the university refectory. When classified by gender, the relationship between the measurements have the structure shown in Figure 10.

The ellipses in this figure reflect the variability of both measured responses and the correlation between them.

**Figure 10:** *Distribution of weight for males and females*

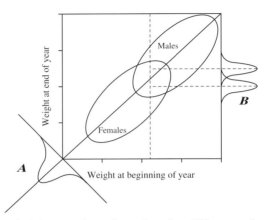

Two statisticians analyse these data for differences in weight gain for males and females. The first statistician makes a comparison of the weight gains between the sexes and concludes that there is no evidence of a correlation between refectory diet and student weight; in particular there is no evidence of a differential effect between the sexes. Neither group shows any regular change.

The second statistician uses ANCOVA and after finding no differences between slopes (a necessary assumption) determines that the differences between intercepts is statistically highly significant. This statistician concludes that the men show a significantly greater weight gain than the women, when proper account is taken of the difference between the sexes.

These two analyses appear to contradict each other. In fact there is no real paradox: the two statisticians are answering different questions, and each is providing the right answer to his respective question, as follows:

*Question:* Is there a difference in the average weight gain between the sexes?

*Answer:* No. The change distributions (A) are identical.

*Question:* Is a male expected to show a greater weight gain than a female, given that they initially of the same weight?

*Answer:* Yes. The conditional distributions given a common initial weight are different (B). This is to be expected because if a male and female are initially of the same weight then either the male is underweight or the female overweight.

The example above, in which the baseline distributions are by definition different, is not appropriate to clinical trials, in which patients are randomly allocated to treatment groups. When using random allocation both approaches are valid and essentially answer the same question. However, the use of baseline measurements is similar to the use of a crossover design, i.e. the use of baselines is like having the patient as their own control, allowing us to remove inter-patient variability and thus gain greater precision in treatment comparisons. Thus we should use ANCOVA in order to increase the precision of treatment comparisons.

# *Q* Why is it necessary to adjust the p-value for multiple comparisons, multiple end-points and interim analyses?

The significance level, as discussed on page 22, is the probability of a false positive, i.e. the probability of declaring that there is a difference between treatments when none exists. In order to answer the question posed above we need to understand under what circumstances the significance level may be altered by the statistical test applied.

Suppose that in analysing a clinical trial it is decided to compare the effects of the two treatments separately in males and females. If two individual tests are carried out at the 5% significance level and find no difference between the treatments, then each test has a 5% chance of giving a false positive result. This also implies that each test has a 95% chance of giving a true negative. Since the tests are independent of each another the probability that both give a true negative is 0.95 x 0.95 = 0.9025, which implies that the probability of making at least one false positive statement is 1 - 0.9025 = 0.0975.

Suppose we follow this procedure: we carry out both tests and if either or both tests give a statistically significant result at the 5% level we declare the treatments are different. If there is truly no difference between the treatments then the true significance level is not 5% as we thought but nearly double that at 0.0975. The effect becomes more pronounced as more subgroups that examined. Table 5 illustrates the relationship between the true significance level and the number of subgroups.

This is the conundrum of multiplicity and it is not restricted to subgroups, but also occurs in the following situations:

*Multiple comparisons*
This arises when two or more treatments are being compared in a single study. In such circumstances there is more than one comparison to be made. For example among three treatments there are three comparisons which can be made, among four treatments there are six comparisons.

**Table 4:** *Relationship between number of subgroups and true significance level*

| Number of subgroups | True significance level |
|:---:|:---:|
| 2 | 0.0975 |
| 3 | 0.1426 |
| 4 | 0.1855 |
| 5 | 0.2262 |
| 6 | 0.2649 |
| 7 | 0.3017 |
| 8 | 0.3366 |
| 9 | 0.3698 |
| 10 | 0.4013 |

*Multiple endpoints*
It is often the case that there is not just a single primary efficacy parameter. If we decide after the data have been analysed that there is a difference between the treatments because one out of a number of end-points is significant the significance level will be increased.

*Multiple looks at data*
The use of interim analyses in clinical research has increased dramatically in the last 20 years. The more frequently we look at the data and carry out tests the more likely it is that we will find a significant result at some stage. Again the true significance level will be increased.

Each of these problems can be resolved by adjusting either the p-value or the significance level which is required to be attained before we declare statistical significance. To illustrate this consider again the subgroup problem and suppose that there are $k$ subgroups. For a nominal significance level of $\alpha$ the true significance level is $1-(1-\alpha)^n$ and if we make this equal to the required level (e.g. 0.05) then we can solve for $\alpha$, the nominal significance level at which each test is to be performed.

For example, if there are six subgroups then we need to solve $0.05 = 1-(1-\alpha)^6$ which gives $\alpha = 0.0085$. So if each individual test is carried out at the 0.0085 significance level the true significance level of making at least one false positive statement is the required 0.05.

There are other ways of doing this:

- Perform a single test between only two treatments, on a single primary efficacy parameter in a pre-defined population of patients. All other tests are regarded as being exploratory and of secondary importance.
- For multiple end-points derive an aggregate end-point based on the individual ones.
- Ignore the problem by reporting all tests whether significant or not. Individual significance levels are never increased; only so-called experiment-wise significance levels are affected by multiplicity.

Unfortunately in drug development the latter approach may not be an option because the regulatory authorities tend to concentrate on experiment-wise significance levels. This restriction is open to debate: why not control a drug development-wise level? Or why not control a company's drug development portfolio-wise level?

# $Q$  Why is the intention-to-treat principle important?

In the perfect clinical trial, every patient entered into the study would meet all the entry criteria, complete the full course of treatment as described in the study protocol, refrain from taking concomitant or rescue medication and provide a full set of data in each and every detail. In practice this never happens!

Problems which may be encountered at the study autopsy include:

- Patients entered who did not meet all the entry criteria.
- Patients who have not been totally compliant or have gaps in their treatment history.
- Patients withdrawn because of intolerable side-effects, no clinical benefit or no longer requiring treatment.
- Patients who have taken concomitant or rescue medication during the study.
- Patients lost to follow-up.

How should patients who are not protocol-compliant be handled?

Traditionally, the primary analysis under non-ideal circumstances would have been a completer, or **per-protocol analysis** which includes only those patients who followed the protocol to the letter. A study is established to compare two or more treatments prescribed in a particular way; the inclusion of data from patients who did not take the treatments according to protocol would bias the resulting treatment estimates. The per-protocol analysis thus reflects a purer estimate of the true treatment difference. The counter argument is that the per-protocol analysis will only provide this purer estimate in certain circumstances. In particular, it requires patients who comply to be equal, in terms of their health status, as those who do not comply. This cannot be true as some have chosen not to comply.

There are many examples which demonstrate how excluding patients from analyses creates bias. The data in Table 5 are derived from a trial which compared surgical and medical therapy for bilateral carotid stenosis.[14]

**Table 5:** *Comparison of surgical and medical treatment for bilateral carotid stenosis*

i) *Excluding in-hospital strokes or deaths:*

| Treatment group | Rate of recurrence/death |
|---|---|
| Surgical | 43/79 = 0.54 |
| Medical | 53/72 = 0.74 |

$\chi^2 = 5.9$, p-value = 0.014

ii) *All patients:*

| Treatment group | Rate of recurrence/death |
|---|---|
| Surgical | 58/94 = 0.62 |
| Medical | 54/73 = 0.74 |

$\chi^2 = 2.80$, p-value = 0.094

The per-protocol analysis (Table 5i) of these data compares the proportions of patients who suffered recurrent transient ischaemic attacks, strokes or death with those patients who were discharged from hospital without suffering a stroke. The p-value of 0.014 indicates that surgical intervention significantly reduces the risk of recurrence or death compared to medical therapy. However in this analysis, 16 patients who suffered a stroke or died in hospital were excluded. Of these, 15 had received surgical intervention and only 1 had received medical therapy.

Another type of analysis, the **intention-to-treat analysis** (table 5ii), includes all patients and increases the p-value to 0.094, which may provide insufficient evidence to conclude that surgery was more beneficial than medical therapy. The intention-to-treat analysis requires that all patients, irrespective of their compliance with protocol, are included in the analysis of the study results. The argument for this approach is that it mirrors actual clinical practice. A clinician treating an individual patient needs to decide how to treat that patient based not on a theoretically ideal circumstance but on the total effect of a treatment strategy, which may need to take account of compliance, the use of rescue medication and other factors.

The intention-to-treat principle raises a number of issues:

1   Some clinicians and statisticians argue for a severe form of the principle in which patients who are known either to have never taken their assigned treatment or who were given the wrong treatment by mistake (this may be discovered if blood samples are taken for compliance monitoring) are analysed as if they had received the original randomly allocated treatment.

2   According to the intention-to-treat principle, if a patient withdraws from the study they will still be included in the analysis. If the outcome variable is death or another major event, then patients who have withdrawn need to be followed up and their outcome ascertained. When the outcome is a continuous measure then some form of imputation is normally used. For example, in an endpoint analysis (also called a last observation carried forward analysis) the last recorded value is used as a final outcome.

3   In the case of continuous outcome measures, the patient may withdraw either before the first dose of the treatment has been taken or before the first post-treatment measurement has been taken. Pragmatically such patients would normally be excluded from the intention-to-treat analysis.

4   The intention-to-treat principle is generally a conservative procedure which reduces treatment differences. However this may not always be appropriate, for example when the objective of a study is to show that two treatments are equivalent.

# Q   What is regression to the mean?

The data in Figure 11 are the scores in the first two rounds of all 156 entrants in the 1995 British Open Golf Championship held at St. Andrews. The vertical and horizontal reference lines are the average first and second round scores (72.7 and 73.9 respectively).

**Figure 11:** *The relationship between first and second round scores in the 1995 British Open Golf Championship*

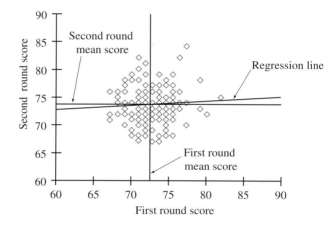

Suppose we consider only individuals who scored between 75 and 77 in the first round. Their mean score in the second round was 74.2, which is closer to the mean of all the second round scores than their mean first round score (75.7) was to the mean of all first round scores. When Francis Galton[15] first observed this in the heights of parents and their children he termed it "regression towards mediocrity". It is now called **regression to the mean**. If we take other groups of individuals with similar first round scores and determine their mean second round scores these pairs of points would lie close to the straight line which is known as the **regression line**.

Why is regression to the mean important in clinical research? The main reason is that individuals are generally chosen to enter studies because they are in some sense extreme. For example, high blood pressure is an indicator of coronary artery disease. Patients with high blood pressure are treated in the expectation of reducing their levels towards normal. However the changes which are seen following treatment may not be due solely to the treatment, and untreated patients will generally show some diminution of effect because of regression to the mean. In other words it is necessary to disentangle the treatment effect from the effect of regression to the mean. The use of concurrent, randomised controls is an appropriate way of doing this.

# *Q* What is meta-analysis?

In simple terms **meta-analysis** is the practice of using statistical methods to combine and quantify the outcomes of a series of studies into a single, pooled analysis. The results of previous studies are extracted from the general medical literature, often using a computer database such as Medline (Ovid). In this definition the emphasis on the use of statistical methods is crucial. In the medical field the scientific review has a long and distinguished history. However, because medical reviews tend to summarise in qualitative rather than quantitative terms and do not utilise statistical approaches, they are generally not viewed as meta-analyses.

**Table 6:** *Incidence of typhoid in inoculated and control individuals*

| Unit | Treatment | Infected | Not Infected | Total |
|------|-----------|----------|--------------|-------|
| 1 | Inoculated | 7 | 21 | 28 |
| | Control | 3 | 10 | 13 |
| 2 | Inoculated | 4 | 55 | 59 |
| | Control | 4 | 21 | 25 |
| 3 | Inoculated | 2 | 10 | 12 |
| | Control | 3 | 35 | 38 |
| 4 | Inoculated | 1 | 19 | 20 |
| | Control | 4 | 30 | 34 |
| 5 | Inoculated | 5 | 16 | 21 |
| | Control | 44 | 66 | 110 |
| 6 | Inoculated | 11 | 76 | 87 |
| | Control | 13 | 34 | 47 |
| 7 | Inoculated | 2 | 68 | 70 |
| | Control | 4 | 8 | 12 |
| 8 | Inoculated | 35 | 1670 | 1705 |
| | Control | 1489 | 9040 | 10529 |
| 9 | Inoculated | 26 | 2509 | 2535 |
| | Control | 257 | 10734 | 10981 |
| 10 | Inoculated | 3 | 197 | 200 |
| | Control | 23 | 524 | 547 |
| 11 | Inoculated | 60 | 640 | 700 |
| | Control | 39 | 455 | 494 |
| 12 | Inoculated | 9 | 293 | 302 |
| | Control | 20 | 224 | 244 |
| 13 | Inoculated | 44 | 44h58 | 4502 |
| | Control | 657 | 25194 | 25851 |
| 14 | Inoculated | 51 | 5948 | 5999 |
| | Control | 731 | 54823 | 54554 |
| 15 | Inoculated | 32 | 4851 | 4883 |
| | Control | 744 | 35211 | 35955 |

The data in Table 6 are taken from an investigation by Pearson[16] into the efficacy of inoculation against typhoid in various units and regiments of the British Army at the turn of the century. Pearson used these data to answer the question of whether there was an association between inoculation and freedom from infection. The modern approach to analysing the data from a single unit would be to determine the odds ratio (see page 32); Pearson worked with the tetrachoric correlation coefficient. The individual estimated odds ratios for the 15 units are shown in Figure 12 with their associated 95% confidence intervals; the individual units are identified and are also clustered.

**Figure 12:** *Meta-analysis of typhoid inoculation data presented in Table 7*

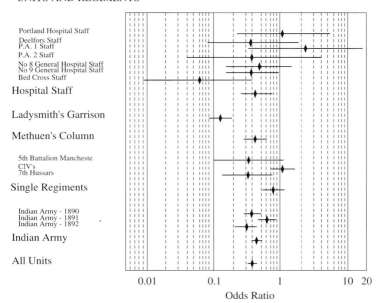

Thus, for example, units 1 to 7 are all hospital staff. Two things are immediately apparent from this figure. First, there is considerable variation between the individual units, a fact noted by Pearson.

Second, the individual estimates themselves have widely different precisions. The statistical problem is how to combine the individual estimates whilst also taking proper account of their individual differing precisions and their heterogeneity. There are two basic statistical approaches to combining such data: a **fixed effects** model and a **random effects** model.

In the fixed effects model it is assumed that there is a single underlying odds ratio and that the differences between the studies are due only to random variation and the differing sample sizes. To illustrate how the estimates are combined, suppose that there are $k$ studies and that each study gives an estimate of the treatment difference and an associated variance which we denote by $\hat{o}_i$ and $v_i$. Then the estimate of the single underlying odds ratio is given by:

$$\hat{O} = \frac{\sum_{i=1}^{k} w_i \hat{O}_i}{\sum_{i=1}^{k} w_i}$$

where $w_i = 1/v_i$. In other words the overall estimate is a weighted average of the individual estimates, where the weight associated with an individual estimate is the reciprocal of its variance. This is intuitively reasonable because a small variance, and hence a large weight, will be given to large studies and the converse to small studies. In Pearson's example we noted that there were considerable differences between individual studies. This may provide evidence that the assumption of a single underlying odds ratio is unreasonable. It is possible to test this assumption.

In the random effects model it is assumed that the individual study parameters themselves have a distribution with some average value $o$ and variance $\sigma^2$. If $\sigma^2$ is known then under this model an estimate of $o$ is given by:

$$\hat{O}^* = \frac{\sum_{i=1}^{k} w^*_i \hat{O}_i}{\sum_{i=1}^{k} w^*_i}$$

where $w^*_i = 1/\{v_i + \sigma^2\}$. In contrast to the fixed effects model, here it is explicitly assumed that there is between-study variation, $\sigma^2$, and that $o$ is an average effect. If there are only a small number of studies the estimate of $\sigma^2$ may be poor. Also large studies do not necessarily gain greater weight because of the appearance of $\sigma^2$ in the individual weights.

What are meta-analyses used for?

- To generate hypotheses. Since their data are extracted from potentially diverse study protocols in the literature, meta-analyses can be extremely useful in providing new hypotheses, especially with regard to subgroups.
- To generate data which are useful in planning new studies. Meta-analyses can provide information on variability, both within and between studies, which is required to determine sample size in new studies.
- To judge consistency across different settings.
- To present results from a series of studies (see Figure 12).
- To increase the precision of the overall estimate.
- Prospectively designed meta-analyses can be helpful in drug development programs.

While they can be extremely useful, meta-analyses have to be treated with caution for the following reasons:

- In prospective, randomised clinical trials most of the planning is aimed at preventing bias. The use of meta-analyses has the potential to re-introduce bias.

- There is the tendency for only positive studies to be published. This is known as publication bias and can lead to an overestimation of the true effect of a treatment if not considered.
- There is the possibility of selection bias if not all studies are utilised.
- Studies which use interim analyses may give rise to biased treatment estimates.
- Meta-analyses may not always be reliable predictors. There is increasing evidence that the results of meta-analyses may conflict with the results from extremely large randomised studies. The reasons for this are not always clear but one cause may be changes over time in treatment practice or patient population.

# *Q* What is Bayesian statistics?

Calculation of a p-value is based on two fundamental principles: (i) probabilities of events are determined prospectively, and (ii) probability is defined in terms of being able to repeatedly sample from a population.

The first principle is based on *deductive logic*. For example, on page 23 we assumed that there was no difference between treatments. Given this assumption, it followed that the chances of a plus or a minus were both 0.5, and therefore that the number of minuses out of 20 pairs followed a Binomial distribution from which the probabilities of any number of minuses out of 20 could be determined. However, many people would argue that what is needed in clinical research is *inductive logic*. Instead of saying 'if the chance of a minus is 0.5 then the probability of 4 minuses out of 20 pairs is 0.000462', inductive logic requires us to make statements of the form 'if we observe 4 minuses out of 20 pairs then the probability that the chance of a minus is 0.5 is for example 0.8'. It is this latter statement which Bayesian statistics aims to provide.

The other key difference between Bayesian statistics and the standard form (generally known as frequentist statistics) is the idea of repeatability. Frequentist statistics views probability as a relative frequency. So, for example, if I were to toss a fair coin many times then approximately half the time it would land on heads, and the more times I tossed the coin the nearer the number of heads would be to one-half. In other words the probability of a head is one half. In Bayesian statistics, however, probability is viewed as a measure of personal belief. Personal beliefs may change as evidence or data accumulate, so if I collect data on the force and angular momentum imparted when the coin is spun then my belief about the likelihood of the coin landing on heads would change (in fact there is experimental evidence to show that knowing both the force and the angular momentum allows us to predict almost perfectly on which face will land). In Bayesian statistics, Bayes' Theorem provides the mechanism for updating beliefs on the basis of new data.

The basic structure of Bayesian statistics is that we start with **prior beliefs** about the phenomenon of interest and these beliefs are quantified in the form of a probability distribution. We then incorporate information from new data, which is termed the **likelihood**, and combine it with our prior beliefs to give the posterior distribution which quantifies **posterior beliefs**.

There have been two major hindrances to the use of Bayesian methods in clinical research:

1    The use of subjective beliefs, i.e. the prior distribution. Many statistcans dislike Bayesian methods because they argue that that are not objective.

2    The practical issue of carrying out the complex calculations required in a Bayesian framework – this problem has been tackled over the last 20 years and viable, practical solutions are now available.

To illustrate the use of Bayesian methods consider the following example. Oxycodone hydrochloride is an opioid analgesic which is commonly used in Finland for treating adult post-operative pain.[17] Studies of oxycodone's pharmacokinetic properties were previously limited to adults but it was decided to study both its pharmacokinetic and pharmacodynamic effects in paediatric patients following ophthalmic surgery.

Clinician A and clinician B are interested in using oxycodone in paediatric patients and believe that the critical parameter is drug clearance rate. Clinician A believes that children are likely to have similar clearance values to adults, in whom previous studies have shown a mean clearance rate of 10 ml/min/kg. Clinician A therefore agrees that a good representation of his prior beliefs is a normal density with mean 10 and standard deviation 2. In contrast, clinician B thinks it likely that owing to the lower body weights of the children the clearance would be larger, approximately 20 ml/min/kg. but that because there is no previous data he is more uncertain about it. He therefore agrees that a good representation of his prior beliefs is a normal density with mean 20 and standard deviation 4. These prior densities are displayed in Figure 13(a).

**Figure 13:** *Example of the use of Bayesian statistics*

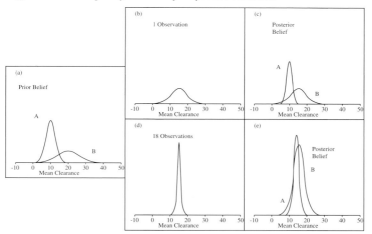

Each clinician is given the result from the first patient, whose clearance was found to be 13.5 ml/min/kg. Suppose that they are both prepared to assume that this measurement is a single realisation of a random variable y which follows a normal distribution with unknown mean μ and standard deviation 4. The shape of the standardised likelihood is shown in Figure 13(b). The posterior densities for clinicians A and B are displayed in Figure 13(c).

From Figures 13(a-c) it can be seen that the beliefs of clinician A have changed little in the light of the data from this single patient; this reflects the fact that strong opinions are likely to be only marginally influenced by a somewhat inaccurate observation. Clinician B, however, has a posterior density which is much closer in form to the likelihood than it is to the prior density. This in turn reflects the fact that individuals with only vague prior beliefs will be greatly influenced by what in effect is an inaccurate observation. Specifically, these observations reflect the fact that the posterior density of clinician A has a mean and standard deviation of 10.7 and 1.8 respectively, which are little changed from the prior values, while the corresponding values for clinician B are 16.8 and 2.8, which show substantial change. The effect of the data has been to move the clinicians' beliefs about paediatric clearance closer to each other; this movement becomes more marked as the amount of data increases.

In the same study, the complete data on 18 patients gave a mean clearance of 15.2 ml/min/kg, which under the assumption of a population standard deviation of 4 has standard deviation $4/\sqrt{18} = 0.94$. The corresponding likelihood is displayed in Figure 13(d) and this is clearly much more concentrated than the likelihood based upon a single observation. The posterior densities for the two clinicians are shown in Figure 13(e). The movement towards a 'consensus' position is now almost complete, and is reflected in the revised posterior means and standard deviations which are 14.3 and 0.85 for clinician A and 15.5 and 0.92 for clinician B respectively.

We can make two inferences from this:

1       If there is considerable data then it is not necessary to know the precise form of prior beliefs.
2       Even apparently substantial prior beliefs may no longer be influential. This is important because of the criticisms of the use of subjective beliefs in Bayesian statistics. If there are sufficient data then the information contained in the data is sufficient to overcome even extremely dogmatic beliefs.

# References

1    Wulff HR, Andersen B, Brandenhoff P, Guttler F. What do doctors know about statistics. Statistics in Medicine, 1987; **6**: 3-10.

2    Barnes CG, Berry H, Carter ME, Downie WW, Fowler PD, Moll MH, Perry JD, Sawaf MS, Wright V. Diclofenac sodium (Voltarol®) and indomethacin: A multicentre comparative study in rheumatoid arthritis and osteoarthritis. Rheumatology and Rehabilitation, 1979; **S2**: 135-146.

3    Braitman LE. Confidence intervals extract clinically useful information from data. Annals of Internal Medicine, 1988; **108**: 296-298.

4    Gardner MJ, Altman DG. Statistics with confidence. London: British Medical Journal, 1989.

5    Hill AB. A short textbook of medical statistics, 11th edition. Edinburgh: Livingstone, 1984.

6    Grieve A, Senn S. Estimating treatment effects in clinical crossover trials. Journal of Biopharmaceutical Statistics, 1998; **8**: 191-243.

7    Freeman PR. The performance of the two-stage analysis of two-treatment, two-period cross-over trials. Statistics in Medicine, 1989; **8**: 1421-1432.

8    Laupacis A, Sackett DL, Roberts RS. An assessment of clinically useful measures of the consequences of treatment. New England Journal of Medicine, 1988; **318**: 1728-1733.

9    Hanley JA. If nothing goes wrong, is everything all right? Journal of the American Medical Association, 1983; **249**: 1743-1745.

10   Altman DG, Bland JM. Absence of evidence is not evidence of absence. British Medical Journal, 1995; **311**: 485.

11    Jones B, Jarvis P, Lewis JA, Ebbutt AF. Trials to assess
      equivalence: the importance of rigorous methods. British
      Medical Journal, 1996; **313**: 36-39.

12    Rikkers LF, Rudman D, Galambos JT, Fulenwider JT,
      Millikan WJ, Kutner M, Smith RB, Salam AA, Sones PJ,
      Warren WD. A randomized, controlled trial of the distal
      splenorenal shunt. The Annals of Surgery, 1978; **188**:
      271-282.

13    Lord FM. A paradox in the interpretation of group compar-
      isons. Psychological Bulletin, 1967; **68**: 304-305.

14    Sackett DL. How to read clinical journals (I) Why to read
      them and how to start reading them critically. Canadian
      Medical Association Journal, 1981; **124**: 555-558.

15    Galton F. Regression towards mediocrity in hereditary
      stature. Journal of the Anthropological Institute, 1886; **15**:
      246-263.

16    Pearson K. Report of certain enteric fever inoculation
      statistics. British Medical Journal, 1904; **3**:1243-1246.

17    Olkkola KT, Hamunen K, Seppälä T, Maunuksela E-L.
      Pharmacokinetics and ventilatory effects of intravenous
      oxycodone in postoperative children. British Journal of
      Clinical Pharmacology, 1994; **38**: 71-76.

18    Lilford RJ, Braunholtz D. The statistical basis of public
      policy: a paradigm shift is due. British Medical Journal,
      1996; **313**: 603-607.

# Questionnaire

Please write to me with your queries regarding any statistical issues in clinical research. I will endeavour to provide a response to all questions received.

AP Grieve

---

**Question(s):**




**Name:**
**Address:**


*Complete this page and return to:*
**Professor A P Grieve**
**c/o Brookwood Medical Publications**
**18-20 Hill Rise**
**Richmond**
**Surrey TW10 6UA**

**Fax: +44 (0)181 332 4610**
**E-mail: managingeditor@bwedit.demon.co.uk**

Brookwood Medical Publication publishes a wide range of handbooks covering the rules and regulations pertaining to the management, performance and monitoring of clinical trials.

Two other Brookwood publications which may be of interest are the *ICH Harmonised Tripartite Guideline for Statistical Principles for Clinical Trials* (1998) and the *Dictionary of Clinical Research* (2nd edition, 1998).

For further information abour Brookwood titles, please contact our Order Administrator by phone +44 (0)181 332 4606, fax +44 (0)181 332 4610 or by e-mail to theresa@brookwood.demon.co.uk.